# THE 1 SYSTEM

## A LIFESTYLE DIET

by
STEVEN FOWLER

## BOOK 1
## *AN INTRODUCTION*

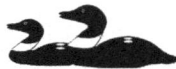

**The 1 System: A Lifestyle Diet** $9.99 USD
"The 1 System" is a practical, reasoned, common sense approach to lifestyle management. "The 1 System" addresses underlying habits contributing to weight gain. Habits that inhibit weight loss and that often result in a myriad of health issues and physical challenges.

**Publisher:** Two Loons Press    **Imprint:** Two Loons Publishing
**Cover Design:** Two Loons Press
All Rights Reserved.
Copyright ©2019 Two Loons Press

## FROM THE PUBLISHER

**Disclaimer**
Neither the Publisher, nor the Author, have control over or responsibility for third-party websites, or any material related to this work that may appear on those websites.

*Printed in the United States of America*
**ISBN:-13 978-1-7324737-5-1**

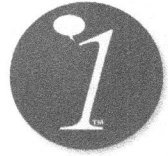

# BULK PURCHASES

"The 1 System" books may be purchased in bulk for educational, business, or sales promotional use; to include bookstores and libraries. For discount and wholesale pricing information, please email:

contact@twoloonspress.com
*Please include "The 1 System Purchases" in the Subject Line*

# FEEDBACK

Send Feedback to:
contact@twoloonspress.com
*Please include "The 1 System Feedback" in the Subject Line*

# INVASION BY PROXY

## A RYAN TATE NOVEL

*Coming Late 2019 or Early 2020*

*An Excerpt...*

It was bad enough to have lost so much, but to endure the discomfort and indignity of the bug-infested swamp was the final straw. Santiago was a man of culture, status, and wealth. A man to be admired and feared, respected and honored.

How could this be happening? Something had gone terribly wrong. After all, he owned politicians, the police, judges, government officials, generals, and the press. His payments for their cooperation and silence should have guaranteed the security of his operations and protected him from this DEA sponsored raid. The Drug Enforcement Administration had gone too far this time. Santiago vowed somebody would die and the filthy Americans would pay dearly for their actions.

As insects ravaged his pampered brown skin, he swore vengeance upon America. His hate rose like bile in the throat. He would get even. Nobody, but nobody, did this to Santiago Monterra. As the morning mist began to rise from his watery hiding place, a vague plan began to form.

# SPY GAMES:
# Inside the Murky World of Corporate Espionage

## A COLA FUGELERE AUTOBIOGRAPHICAL NOVEL

*Available on Amazon*
*(Print and Kindle Versions)*

*An Excerpt...*

I was in Washington D.C. conducting operations relating to a technology transfer. The operation had gone well and finished on a high note. Team members split up and departed the area quickly. One flew out of Baltimore, and another took the train to NY. Ryan caught a bus to North Carolina, where he caught a flight out of Charlotte Douglas International Airport. A colleague, not directly involved with the operation, waited 140 miles away in Frostburg, Maryland. He was scheduled to pick me up in front of Ford's Theater at midnight and drive all night to Milwaukee for my flight to San Jose, so I could deliver the $225,000.00 USB.

As I was waiting for my ride, I decided to enjoy an adult beverage at a dark, quiet venue near the White House. While there I overheard a young woman utter a most regrettable statement. I immediately took a pen from my pocket and memorialized her words. She said, "You don't get it. I'm advancing my career. I'm connected, moving forward, and I'm destined to impact history. I will become part of the history of D.C., this nation, this world. Whatever it takes to succeed. It'll happen, and God help anyone who gets in my way. Get in my way and I'll run you over. I WILL SUCCEED AT ANY COST!"

She was on Cola's payroll three months later.

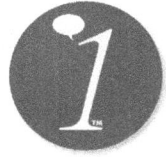

# FROM THE AUTHOR

**General Disclaimer**
This book series employs common sense solutions to portion control and overeating. These are neither medical books nor an attempt to override sound medical advice. Moreover, they are not intended to replace specific dietary plans designed by professionals for individuals based on the physical, mental, nutritional, or medical needs of the reader.

While followers of these books may enjoy weight loss in many, if not most, cases, "The 1 System" is not intended to serve as a temporary weight loss regimen. Readers are encouraged to use the general guides in this series to assist them to better manage food intake and body mass by modifying their lifestyles in positive ways.

**Specific Disclaimer**
Consult your physician before you modify your eating habits. You should also discuss lifestyle modifications with your doctor before you begin this, or any other, diet or exercise program.

This author and the publisher are not providing medical advice in these books. We are not medical doctors and are not making medical claims in this series. See your physician before following any of the suggestions found within these pages.

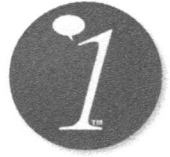

# THANK YOU

Thank you for choosing "The 1 System." We really want to help you overcome lifestyle challenges impacting the quality of your life.

We developed this lifestyle approach to diet because we recognize many popular methods for weight loss aren't the answer for most people. Moreover, after a temporary loss in weight, most weight loss programs result in additional weight gain, cyclical efforts, and loss of self-esteem.

Weight loss not the primary goal of "The 1 System's" practical approach to living. It is, however, a wonderful side benefit that will be enjoyed by many, if not most, people who embrace "The 1 System." We hope to guide you in discarding bad habits. We want to help you develop new routines that should, ultimately, result in a new, healthier, slimmer, and better you.

# PREORDERING

"The 1 System" Book 2 is scheduled for publication by Two Loons Press in Late 2019. Pre-Ordering will be available for this book.

# DEDICATION

This series is dedicated to everyone who struggles daily to gain meaningful control of their lives. In that, we hope the lifestyle habits introduced in this series will offer a measure of assistance for you in achieving your goals.

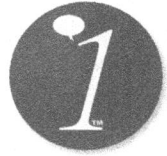

# INTRODUCTION

Hello. I'm Steven Fowler. I firmly believe "The 1 System" can work for most people who adopt the positive habits outlined in this series. Remember, you are the 1 person who can choose to make a real difference in your life and health.

Every reader should consult their physician prior to the start of any diet or exercise program.

My wife of many years believes I should weigh more than 400 pounds. However, my weight is less than ½ that. That said, she is correct. She recognizes my powerful gluttonous traits. Why stop at 1 cheeseburger, when there are 2 more on the grill that nobody's going to eat? What's wrong with eating an entire roasted chicken, when I'm not yet satisfied; besides it will just go to waste (or, more accurately, "to my waist").

You think I'm kidding? I'm deadly serious. I cannot count how many times I've eaten more than 40 Hot (Buffalo) Wings at a sitting. I've also consumed dozens of escargot during a single meal, and on one occasion ate more than 40 of the slimy slugs. I've eaten entire roasted chickens more times than I can begin to count. Pizza? There are more slices in the box. Why stop?

Speaking of pizza. Pizza was the genesis for "The 1 System." I realized I was eating extra large pizzas all by myself, during a period when I was working out of town and staying in a tiny apartment without my family. I was pigging out, 1 slice at a time. Those single slices led me to consider the number 1.

I looked at an empty pizza box, then opened the freezer. The freezer had plenty of space I could have used to store that last piece of pizza that I really didn't need. I decided the next time I had pizza, I'd freeze the last slice as a future snack.

The next time I pigged out on a huge pizza, I placed the last slice in a plastic bag and put it in the freezer compartment. Then I belched and realized I shouldn't have eaten that second to the last slice. That piece could have been frozen as well. I vowed to eat 1 less slice the next time I had pizza.

That happened repeatedly. I ate 1 less slice each time. I finally reached a point where I was eating a single slice of pizza each pizza night, and saving many more slices for future consumption. It was all about 1.

After a time I found pounds melting off my body, 1 pound at a time; all the while I was spending much less on food. I realized there was power in the number 1 when it came to how I consume food. I took it to the next level.

Why eat 1 whole roasted chicken, when I would be well satisfied with 1 chicken breast? Over the next few months, I found myself using Logic + 1 to find my way to better eating and improved health. I quickly discovered the power in that formula.

I was in pretty good shape when I turned 40. When I was 49 I set a goal of turning 50; in far better shape than I was on my 40th birthday. I met that goal, thanks to "The 1 System."

**"The Power of 1"**
Without "The 1 System," I would be that round 400-pound man my bride knows could be me. I believe The Power of 1 has saved me. I've been considering putting my "1" tactics, tips, tools, and tricks into a book for more than a dozen years. *It's time to share The Power of 1 with others!*

I hope and trust YOU, and many others, will benefit from "The 1 System: A Lifestyle Diet."

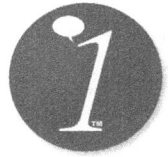

# FOREWORD
## by
## Harry L. Greene II MD

As a specialist in Preventive Medicine, over the past twenty years I have noted that almost any reasonable, scientifically supported, weight loss program will work during the period of time it is assiduously followed.

"The 1 System's" developer, Steven Fowler, recognizes that a 90% relapse rate is commonplace during the maintenance period of most diet plans. Mr. Fowler developed "The 1 System" with the understanding that most dieters regain lost weight; in some cases gaining even more. That recognition led him to the development of a lifestyle diet program designed to overcome those issues.

"The 1 System" teaches us intelligent eating must become an ingrained habit. Its tools are designed to assist followers beyond those offered by common short term diet plans, programs that encourage eating commercially prepared weight loss food, or methods requiring convening with others who use situational support to remain on the program.

Mr. Fowler is correct. One must embrace and incorporate lifestyle changes, and reflect them consistently in daily choices. Only then will success be yours.

As part of my Preventive Medicine Fellowship at Stanford in 1989, I visited and/or enrolled in WEIGHT WATCHERS and Jenny Craig, along with several others. They all worked while under observation, but the relapse rate was near 100% unless you kept going to counseling or group therapy. Rarely someone would figure it out and succeed for a reasonable life-changing period of time. "The 1 System" holds great promise in this area.

Harry L. Greene II MD

*Dr. Greene spent 34 years in medicine. His various postings include the Sydney Farber Cancer Institute, Harvard Medical School, University of Massachusetts (Primary Care and Preventive Medicine), Stanford University, and the University of Arizona. He also served as Chief Executive Officer of the Massachusetts Medical Society (17,000 doctors) and Publisher of The New England Journal of Medicine. Dr. Greene has edited or co-edited 7 medical textbooks, and worked under grants from the Bill and Melinda Gates Foundation; translating his work into Russian, for primary care physicians in that nation.*

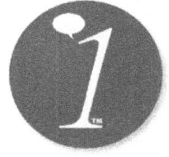

# A SPECIAL ACKNOWLEDGMENT

### by Steven Fowler
Author and Creator of "The 1 System"

I'd like to take a moment and thank my dear friend, Dr. Harry L. Greene, for his many acts of kindness in the time I've known him.

He is a true gentleman of the highest caliber. Selfless to the core. I'm honored to know him and thrilled with the opportunities I've had to learn from this special mentor of mine. I appreciate him more than he could ever know and value every moment we spend together. His continual support and encouragement provides this author with resolve and a desire to better myself at every turn.

I'm especially honored by his willingness to endorse "The 1 System" and contribute to the manuscript in various ways.

My last book exceeded 600 pages and, to my knowledge, Dr. Greene was the very first person to read the entire book. His enthusiasm for "SPY GAMES: Inside the Murky World of Corporate Espionage" is contagious and certainly contributed to that book's success.

Thank you "Mo" for all you do for Tracey and me. Your efforts on my behalf are certainly appreciated. You and your wife, Linda, are rare gifts. You bless our lives by just being you.

I eagerly anticipate further collaborative opportunities with you,

Steve...

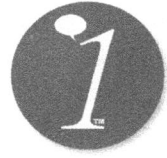

# THE 1 SYSTEM
## A LIFESTYLE DIET

by
STEVEN FOWLER

## BOOK 1
### *AN INTRODUCTION*

**IMPORTANT NOTE**

Two Loons Press and Steven Fowler purposely designed the paperback version with large areas of lined space in this book; intended for your use. We trust and hope you'll use it often to memorialize your thoughts, and for future reference.

We encourage followers to keep a pen or pencil handy to jot down notes, thoughts, "1 ideas" of your own design, goals, plans, etc... Use that space to plan, journal, and record your habit modification plans and goals.

*Fad Diets <u>DO NOT</u> Work!*

*"Hey, did you hear about the new diet everybody's talking about?"*

Throughout this book we will continually repeat the message that fad diets do not, will not, and cannot work in the long term.

The message is that important.

## AGE APPROPRIATE WEIGHT

"We should live with an appropriate weight for our height and age."

~Harry L. Greene II MD

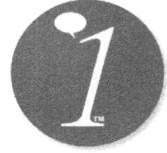

# WHAT IS A DIET IN THE
# THE 1 SYSTEM UNIVERSE?

# *1*

*Not, #2*

**Diet can be defined as:**

1.  Normal consumption
2.  Specific foods and liquids consumed for specific purposes (such as weight loss or weight management).

Which definition best describes what you think of when you hear the word: DIET? Like most people, your first thought is probably #2 above.

If more people would pay better attention to and adjust their usual habitual "diet" (#1 above), rather than engaging in temporary weight loss efforts commonly referred to as temporary or fad diets (#2 above), we would be healthier people carrying fewer pounds.

# *ATTENTION!*

**"The 1 System"
isn't just for people
with current weight loss needs.**

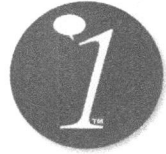

# WARNING!

# 1

## Important Consideration for Young Thin People

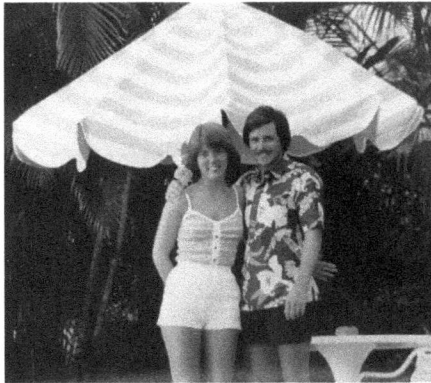

**Tracey and Steven Fowler**

Young people don't think it will happen to them. We certainly didn't.

One day, many who are now young and thin, will have weight management issues. Taken on our wedding day, this is a photo of

*Intended for Reader Use*

# THE 1 SYSTEM

Tracey and me. I'm sure neither of us would have guessed on that day that we'd eventually consider and/or fret about our weight, in one manner or another, nearly every day as we ventured into middle age. I believe to the core of my being, if I would have adopted "The 1 System" when I was young and thin, my life would have even better.

Our two children have been a real blessing. After they were born, Tracey remained thin. She was always on the thin side. Then we transitioned through our 30's. Things began to change. When she and I crossed into our 40's, the change continued.

Over the years, insidious sneaky fat cells began to accumulate on both of us. Once those pesky adipocytes (fat cells) took hold, they became more and more difficult to manage.

> *We know what we are,*
> *but know not what we may become.*
> *- William Shakespeare*

Shakespeare only revealed part of the matter. We knew we weren't overweight on our wedding day, but good old William didn't tell us what would become of those firm, lean bodies of ours.

I thought of our two younger slimmer bodies shortly before "The 1 System" was published. A young woman we know chided me when I offered to send her a signed copy of the printed version of my book. Some months ago a very slim "K" gave birth to her first child. That new mother was joking (I hope) and asked, "Are you telling me I haven't lost all the baby weight yet?"

Trying to tactfully dig myself out of the hole I'd created, I responded with, "I'm not very smart, but I am smarter than that. I like living. Who knows... Perhaps a chubby friend of yours might see 'The 1 System' sitting on your coffee table and rush to buy a thousand copies."

# STEVEN FOWLER

*Intended for Reader Use*

_____

_____

_____

_____

_____

_____

_____

_____

_____

_____

_____

_____

_____

_____

_____

_____

After mulling the matter over for a while, I recalled something said by Emerson.

> *The only person you are destined to become,*
> *is the person you choose to be.*
> *- Ralph Waldo Emerson*

Emerson was correct. However, as a young person, I never stopped to consider the wisdom of his words in the context of weight management as I aged. I never consciously regarded weight choices as something I should address while still slim. I probably thought I'd address weight issues if and when weight became a problem.

I've learned weight is generally a symptom of three underlying problems — lethargy, quantity, and type (detailed in the next section); in one combination or another. If eating and physical activity habits in my twenties were better and more in line with "The 1 System," I doubt those 3 or 4 extra additional pounds in my 30's would have materialized. The extra dozen pounds discovered in my 40's are clearly related to bad eating habits I adopted in my 20's.

Face it, twenty-year-old kids can usually get away with poor eating habits and food binges without too many short term problems. However, add ten years to the person, and things begin to change. Add another decade. Cause and effect changes entirely. Poor eating habits reveal themselves in unflattering unhealthy ways.

The same pizza night twenty years ago affected my body much differently than it would today. While in college I really enjoyed Hot Fudge Sundaes, with extra nuts and

*Intended for Reader Use*

_____

_____

_____

_____

_____

_____

_____

_____

_____

_____

_____

_____

_____

_____

_____

fudge. Today that awesome treat would cost my body in a number of disturbing ways.

If I hadn't adopted "The 1 System" in my 40's, I would be that 400 pound man my wife knows could be me. Without "The 1 System" I believe I would still be over-indulging and harming myself by eating too much pizza, too many ice cream treats, and stuffing myself with other unhealthy tasty items on a daily basis.

In short, I believe young people would benefit by adopting the precepts presented in "The 1 System" while they are still young. Eating smart when young and thin, and developing good healthy eating habits earlier in life, will sustain young people as they transition through the aging process. It'll reduce their struggles, keep them in comfortable clothing longer, and serve their health well.

*Face it. Fad diets don't work!*

Fad diets generally hype weight loss in days or weeks. They'll tell you it's easy. By now you know better. Most followers ultimately fail to achieve their goals and ask why.

*Why am I still fat?*
*Why did my weight return?*
*Why can't I keep my weight off?*

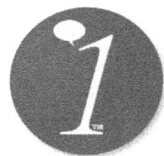

# WHY?

# 1

### Set of Facts You Already Know

**Why am I overweight?**
The underlying issues resulting in weight problems for most people generally fall into one or more of the following three categories:

1. Lethargy: You Are Too Sedentary
2. Quantity: You Eat Too Much
3. Type: You Eat Bad Stuff

Some people eat well, but don't move. Others move frequently, but eat too much of the wrong thing. Some simply overeat. For many, it's all three.

**Lethargy**
You cannot burn calories and fat efficiently if you remain inactive. You'll be happy to know that too much activity can be dangerous and is often counterproductive. You don't have to kill yourself at the gym. Just move. Most people need to move more.

# STEVEN FOWLER

*Intended for Reader Use*

## Quantity

It's a no-brainer. Most of you know, if you consume more than your body will burn, you'll gain weight.

## Type

What types of food are making you fat? Foods come in many varieties and can affect you in various way that may surprise you; resulting in weight gain.

### FOOD LABELS

"The Food and Drug Administration (FDA) has tried to help us by requiring the calories and components of food placed on an easy to read label to the side, or back, of packaged food. Recently they have extended this labeling to restaurant menus."

~Harry L. Greene II MD

*Ever Consider Walking Across the Continent?*

*Like Modifying Habits…*
*You Take 1 Step At A Time*

## GRADUAL CHANGES

"The late Robert Sweetgall walked across North America to demonstrate the comfort and durability of Rockport shoes. You don't have to walk across America. Just walk a little further every day."
~Harry L. Greene II MD

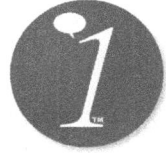

# TACTICS, TIPS, TOOLS, & TRICKS

## 1
### Step At A Time

THE 1 SYSTEM series presents a unique approach to lifestyle habit modification. We first assist you in identifying and addressing your bad habits in Book 1: The Introduction.

It is essential for followers to understand their strengths, weaknesses, subconscious habits, and much much more if they want to have a fighting chance in achieving and maintaining their goals.

Lifestyle identification is a critical need. If you cannot readily identify the problem, then you're more likely to ignore effective solutions.

The second and following books are designed to reveal tactics, tips, tools, and tricks (4T's) that have been successfully adopted by the readers of Book 1.

## EXERCISE

"In 1978 I was impressed when a colleague of mine ran and completed the Boston Marathon. It seemed like a very long way.

"At the time I was Chief Resident at Brigham and Women's Hospital in Boston. I wanted to try running the marathon myself, but I feared I wouldn't stick with it... so I teamed up with one of the residents named Gail Brown.

"Every night we donned our running shoes and went out for a run, adding a block or two every time. On weekends we scheduled a longer run if we had free time. Sometimes I didn't feel like it and sometimes (rarely) she didn't feel like it, but we persisted.
"On Patriot's Day in 1978 we completed the Boston Marathon in slightly over 4 hours. We had a plan and we stuck to it.

"In 1978 everyone seemed to be enchanted with Eastern Philosophy. Our mantra was, 'The journey of a thousand miles begins with a single step!' It seems trite now, but still relevant."

~Harry L. Greene II MD

**NOTE**: *Readers will be able to present their own 1's on our website. Their recommendations will be presented in the following manner:*

### SERVING

1 serving only. The practice of returning for second and third servings is commonplace and detrimental.

Don't refill your plate. A single serving is normally sufficient for your nutritional needs if your diet is well balanced and supplemented by a good multivitamin.
Tatum C.
Mesa, Arizona

## BOOK 1
### "THE 1 SYSTEM: A Lifestyle Diet - An Introduction"
Book 1 is designed to help readers better understand and recognize bad eating habits, and to understand that any approach to habit modification should be taken 1 step at a time. As the title indicates, it is an introduction; the first step to a new you.

This book offers followers a variety of effective tactics tips, tools, and tricks designed to assist them in developing their own approach to "The 1 System" and their need to overcome counterproductive lifestyle habits.

## BOOK 2
### "THE 1 SYSTEM: A Lifestyle Diet – Reader Recommendations"
Book 2 will contain a series of helpful tactics tips, tools, and tricks developed by successful followers of "The 1 System."

*A Chemist Might Look at Dieting Like This:*

**Heat Released by Burning Fat:**

$$E_h = cM_w\Delta T$$

**A Calorie is:**
**A Unit of Energy**

**Per Calorie Variables in Food:**
**<u>Measurement: Grams</u>**

| | |
|---:|:---|
| Carbohydrate: | 4 Calories |
| Protein: | 4 Calories |
| Fat: | 9 Calories |

**Burn > Consumption = Dieting**

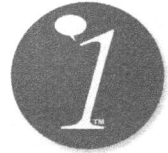

# UNDERSTANDING LABELS AND CALORIES

*1*

**Fundamental Fact**
**YOU NEED TO READ AND UNDERSTAND FOOD LABELS**

### Short and Sweet

Food contain energy (calories). If you consume more calories than you burn, excess energy is stored by your body in fatty cells. Fat cells increase your bulk. Fat cells make you fat.

### Labels

We encourage you to become familiar with food labels. If they're unfamiliar to you, keep reading them. In no time at all you'll begin to understand and will take time to view labels while shopping.

Food labels and becoming familiar with calories isn't rocket science. Teaching readers all about food labels and calories is outside the scope of this book. There are many good resources online to assist novices who choose to learn more about this subject.

We offer you the following from the FDA's website:

> **General Guide to Calories**
>     40 Calories is low
>     100 Calories is moderate
>     400 Calories or more is high
>
> The General Guide to Calories provides a general reference for calories when you look at a Nutrition Facts label.
>
> This guide is based on a 2,000 calorie diet.
>
> **Eating too many calories per day is linked to overweight and obesity.**

## NOT KNOWING THE BASICS CAN LEAD TO A FATTER YOU

Here's a real life example of someone I personally know who blew her diet because she didn't understand calories and other food basics:

"Donna" was on a weight loss program that offered substitution options for followers. For example, a dieter might substitute fat free yogurt for a dish that calls for sour cream.

"Donna" didn't follow, care about, understand, or appreciate just how sugar, fat, and other ingredients would impact her diet. In her case, ignorance was both bliss and counterproductive.

My wife, Tracey, was mentoring "Donna" in her dieting efforts. Tracey dropped by to see her friend one afternoon and was shocked to see her very overweight friend eating ice cream.

"What are you doing? You can't have ice cream on your diet!"

"Donna" replied she was following the diet's substitution plan. The woman told Tracey she wasn't in the mood for milk that afternoon. "Donna" decided to substitute 1 cup of ice cream for the 1 cup of milk that she was scheduled to drink.

There's a lesson in "Donna's" error for everyone who decides to modify their dietary intake:

## KNOW WHAT'S GOING INTO YOUR BODY
## AND
## HOW IT MAY IMPACT YOUR HEALTH & WEIGHT

**The Good, the Bad, and the Ugly**
We want everyone to succeed with "The 1 System." To do that, readers need to understand food basics. If the following information is news to you (something you didn't know/realize), I suggest you study the basics of food and nutrition as part of adopting a new dietary lifestyle.

- Did you know bananas are loaded with sugar?
- Did you know avocados are filled with fat? Good fat?
- Did you know granola may be expanding your waistline?
- Did you know grocery stores breakfast food aisles are loaded with sugar-filled processed foods?
- Did you know many power bars and "healthy" snack foods are filled with sugar and refined carbohydrates?
- Did you know carrots are fat-free?
- Did you know white bread can play havoc with your blood sugar levels and result in you overeating?
- Did you know most fruit juices are loaded with sugar and are generally unhealthy additions to your diet?
- Did you know that fructose is a sugar?

*Change vs. More of the Same*

*Face it. Fad diets don't work!*

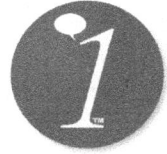

# THE MRL LIFESTYLE

## 1

**Foundational Truth About "The 1 System"**

"The 1 System's" MRL Lifestyle approach to better living resides in a single word: **HABIT.**

**Habit can be defined as:**

1. A repetitious activity in the mind, reflected in the body
2. Behaviors consistent with prior behaviors
3. An automatic response based on repetition
4. Something performed easily, because doing so is normal
5. Typical behavior for the person doing it

Most reasonable people agree that inactivity and poor eating habits, as opposed to genetic influences, are the reasons so many people are overweight. "The 1 System" addresses counterproductive dietary and sedentary habits; and presents reasonable alternatives for healthier lifestyles and weight reduction.

We believe "The 1 System" will work for most who adopt our lifestyle approach to managing their bodies and food consumption.

## Habit Modification
Habits are not hardwired into our bodies or brains, but are nevertheless difficult to change.

"The 1 System's" MRL Lifestyle Diet tools and techniques are designed to assist you in successfully embracing modifications to your lifestyle so that bad habits can become former habits.

# MRL?
*We know, you're curious about the meaning of MRL.*

MRL is an acronym for Modification, Reinforcement, and Listening. Let me explain.

## M = Modification
Any expectation of reducing your weight and keeping lost pounds from returning MUST involve the modification of your dietary habits and/or an increase in your exercise. Old habits made your weight gain possible. New and better habits are critical to losing weight and keeping it off.

### SEEKING TOOLS FOR YOUR CIRCUMSTANCES

> "When I couldn't run during my marathon training, I made a conscious effort to use the stairs as I went around the hospital."
>
> ~Harry L. Greene II MD

## R = Reinforcement
Weight loss efforts and weight maintenance desires will easily fail if your efforts to adopt new healthier habits aren't continually

reinforced. "The 1 System," by design, will assist you by providing many avenues for continual reinforcement.

## L = Listening

Any person who struggles with weight issues MUST learn to listen and respond to those subtle and not so subtle messages being sent by our bodies. Many people will try to ignore a screaming body, telling them, "I'm stuffed!" They will continue shoveling food into their mouths. Most overweight people do not actively "listen" to what their bodies or common sense are telling them. "The 1 System" provides tools to assist you in listening and responding to your body.

Do you listen to your body? Our bodies are very effective in sending important signals and work hard to tell us what we need to hear. Unfortunately, many individuals struggling with weight issues have learned to tune out messages their body is sending.

### WHO ARE YOU LISTENING TO?

"Sometimes people listen to others. You want the person who prepared the food to know you liked it. So you have that additional helping to show your appreciation. Listen you your body, not others!"
~Harry L. Greene II MD

## BREAKING THE MOLD

"The 1 System's" MRL Lifestyle Diet offers you a variety of tools in your quest to break old destructive habits; habits that resulted in the excess girth you'd like to shed. The primary tool in this approach is "The Power of 1." The purpose of 1 is to consciously remind you of your obligation to modify food intake and increase physical activity. Using these tools on a regular basis should assist most readers in positive lifestyle modifications and help develop better habits.

*Don't Forget Your Health!*

*Fad diets can be dangerous!*

## FAD DIETS AND POPULAR PROGRAMS

"Some fad diets can be unhealthy and geared toward immediate weight loss at the expense of your health.

"Popular weight loss programs WEIGHT WATCHERS, Jenny Craig, and NUTRISYSTEM have been cleared by nutritionists and physicians. I do not consider them unhealthy fad diets.

"Most weight loss programs just don't work during the post-diet Maintenance Period.*"

~Harry L. Greene II MD

*Maintenance Period explained:
That period after the "diet" is "over."*

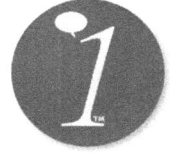

# IN A WORD

## 1

### General Truth

### When It Comes To Eating,
### High Quantity & High Quality Are Polar Opposites

**Quantity**

"The 1 System's" MRL techniques do not focus reader attention on pumping iron, killing oneself on exercise equipment, or running marathons. "The 1 System" knows measuring calories, carbohydrates, and body fat can be both time consuming and frustrating. While all of these things may be of some value to readers, we recognize the primary problem is:

### Q-U-A-N-T-I-T-Y

Most people simply eat too much and consume unnecessary quantities of the wrong things. The techniques offered in "The 1 System's" MRL will assist readers seeking to reduce food intake to reasonable levels.

### *Is It Up To Me?*

*YOU can make a difference in your
health, weight, and eating habits.*

Don't rely on others to do it for you.
Yes, it's up to you.

## THE KEY PLAYER

"If there are others in your life who encourage you, by all means use them; but the key player in this game is YOU!"

~Harry L. Greene II MD

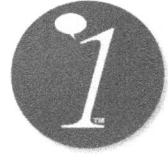

# MY "TREAT ME" HABIT

# 1

## Deviation Leads To Another

**Mission creep...**

We have all developed habits on a subconscious level that dictate our daily actions and activities. I have tried, for example, to watch my fat and cholesterol intake for the past 30 years. Unfortunately, many years ago I adopted certain exceptions to my self imposed rules as part of a "Treat Me" reward for being faithful in reducing my overall fat intake. One of those exceptions included the rare treat of tamales prepared with lard at my favorite Mexican restaurant.

Over the years, I found myself scheduling more and more business and personal meetings at that restaurant. Without realizing it, I had radically increased my fat intake. My once rare treat became a thrice weekly (or more) event. Out of habit and without thinking, I ordered my standard fare without looking at the menu and seeking a healthier alternative.

*Advertisers encourage consumers to*

# Super Size

*They are interested in your money.*

**We encourage readers to**
Down Size

*We are interested in your health,*
*quality of life, and peace of mind.*

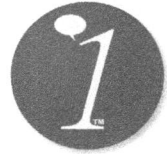

# SUBCONSCIOUS HABITS

## 1

### Example of Counterproductive Subconscious Activities

**Guilty!**

I know some people who will walk into their kitchen, open the refrigerator, take out a soda, drink it until gone, throw the can away, and one hour later not remember they'd even had the soda. They will do this repeatedly day after day. Before developing "The 1 System," I performed this act almost daily, with many kinds of food and drink.

We see parallels in smokers. Smokers will purchase a carton of cigarettes, and before they know it, the carton is empty. Most don't realize how much they've been smoking until long after most of the cigarettes are gone. Such habits are described effectively by Webster's as acts "repeated so often by an individual that it has become automatic with him." Automatic actions generally take place on the subconscious level.

People must consciously watch and review their actions, over extended periods, in order to develop new habits designed to replace old unhealthy habits. Those engaged in such lifestyle

33

*Intended for Reader Use*

modifications need to employ the use of special tools to avoid falling back into old and destructive habits. Reminders, alerts, and other techniques are critical for those engaging in any serious effort to modify automatic subconscious actions.

## Let "1" be your reminder.

### THE INSIDIOUS TELEVISION

"I encourage readers of Steven Fowler's 'The 1 System' to count the number of food advertisements you see during an evening watching television. It's disgusting how many pitches there are for food after dinnertime. These marketing efforts are often followed by TV watchers taking a trip to the refrigerator!"

~Harry L. Greene II MD

*Fad diets do not work*

*"I'm on a diet to lose weight and*
*cannot wait until this diet is over!"*

WHY DIET TEMPORARILY?
Do you really want to regain
the pounds you just lost?

## CONSIDER COMBINING PROGRAMS

"In psychology there is a concept called self-effacing. It is an internally held concept that you CAN do this or you CAN'T do this. Most of the time whichever of these views you hold... you will be right.

"If you believe Jenny Craig or NUTRISYSTEM will work for you... Try it.

But, when the diet is over, transfer to Steven Fowler's 'The 1 System' Lifestyle Diet for success and sustained progress."

~Harry L. Greene II MD

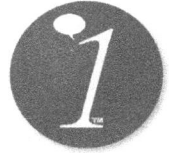

# A TEMPORARY FIX

# 1
## Important Factoid About Fad Diets

By definition, a fad is a fantasy that only lasts for a short time. I like to refer to it as a "short-lived craze that will last about as long as your weight loss efforts."

*Fad diets are unhelpful and will achieve only temporary weight loss most of the time, for most dieters.*

A fad diet is a form, or method, of food consumption that only lasts for a short period of time. In fact, most people only remain on a diet for a little while, until they reach certain goals. Upon completion of the diet, most will resume their previous (abnormal) eating habits and rapidly return to, and exceed, their pre-diet weight. This approach to weight management is cyclical, unhealthy, and unmistakably counterproductive.

*"Going For Seconds Can't Hurt"*
## Wrong!

If you purchased this book, you
know you need to lose weight.
*Right?*

**Don't go for that 2$^{nd}$ portion.
This isn't The 2 System!**

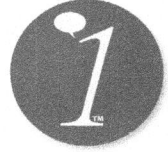

# TEMPORARY DIETING DOESN'T WORK

# *1*

**Important Fact**

**Going on a diet does not work.
Don't allow anyone to convince you otherwise.
It's a false promise!**

As the world gets fatter, more diet books are sold. Yet, fatty pounds continue to accumulate on good old planet earth.

Don't buy into the hype. Don't sign on to the latest dieting fad.

**AGAIN...
TEMPORARY DIETS DO NOT WORK!!!**

*If At First You Don't Succeed*

*Try Try Again!*

## A FRESH START

> "Failure or a mistake is simply a chance to begin again more intelligently."
>
> ~Harry L. Greene II MD

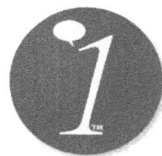

# I FELL OFF MY DIET!

## 1
### Important Perspective

"The 1 System" has some novel responses and perspectives when we hear someone say, "I fell off my diet!"

In a word: SO?
In a few words: GET BACK ON!

This author blows it every now and then (more often that I'd like to admit). So I might have eaten like a pig last night. Should that excuse a decision to eat a 6 Egg Cheese and Sausage Omelet this morning? NO! Should I eat a Hot Fudge Sundae this afternoon? Again, NO!

It means I deviated from my chosen lifestyle, but that doesn't make the deviation permanent or an excuse to drop "The 1 System." Let each day stand on its own. Do your level best each day to focus on doing that which is necessary to solidify and honor your newfound habits. Over time those "fell off my diet" incidents will, hopefully, melt away. We trust that will be followed by your excess weight.

*Ecclesiastes 1:9 (NIV)*
*What has been will be again,*
*what has been done will be done again;*
*there is nothing new*
*under the sun.*

*Proverbs 23:2*
*...and put a knife to your throat if*
*you are given to gluttony.*

### IMPORTANT NOTE
"The 1 System" is NOT recommending anyone use the "knife to your throat" approach. We are simply pointing out there's a dangerous, self-destructive nature to gluttony.

## YOU ARE IN CHARGE OF YOUR PROGRESS

> "You know what isn't working. The symbolic knife is yours. That which is impairing your progress, should be cut out."
>
> ~Harry L. Greene II MD

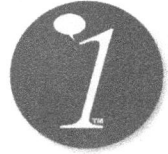

# GLUTTONY IS NOTHING NEW

# 1

## Lesson About Gluttony

### Excerpts from
### "The Diary of a Country Parson"

The following excerpts were contained in the personal diary of Reverend James Woodforde of Somerset, England. These specific passages were written in 1774, when Rev. Woodford was 34 years old. The diary, titled "The Diary of a Country Parson," was first published in 1924, more than 100 years after his death.

*NOTE: We opted to leave spelling and other issues untouched.*

**January 26**
he had a very elegant dinner. The dinner was as follows. First course Cod and Oyster Sauce, Rost Beef, Tongue and boiled Chicken, Peas, Soups and Roots. The second course a boiled Turkey by mistake of the Manciple, which should have been rested, a brace [2] of Partridges rested, 4 Snipes and some Larkes rested, also an orange pudding, syllabubs and jellies, Madeira and Port Wines to Drink and a dish of Fruit.

**April 20**
Mr. Bowerbank, Mr. Shackleford, Mr. Mines, Mr Rigby, Mr. Selstone, Mr. Morris, and Mr. Rawbone dined with us there Mr. NichoUs was ill and could not come, and Mr. Cooke not in town. We had

a very elegant dinner. The first course was, part of a large Cod, a Chine of Mutton, some Soup, a Chicken Pye, Puddings and Roots etc. Second course, Pidgeons and Asparagus, a Fillet of Veal with Mushrooms and high Sauce with it, rested Sweetbreads, hot Lobster, Apricot Tart and in the middle a Pyramid of Syllabubs and Jelhes. We had a Desert of Fruit after Dinner, and Madeira, white Port and red to drink as Wine. We were all very cheerful and merry.

## June 8
Mr. and Mrs. Custance and Mr. du Quesne dined and spent the afternoon with us and stayed till 8 o'clock in the evening. I gave them for dinner, a Couple of Chicken boiled and a Tongue, a Leg of Mutton boiled and Capers and Batter Pudding for the first Course, Second, a couple of Ducks rested and green Peas,
some Artichokes, Tarts and Blancmange. After dinner, Almonds and Raisins, Oranges and Strawberries. Mountain and Port Wines. Peas and Strawbernes the first gathered this year by me. We spent a veiy agreeable day, and all well pleased and merry.

## July yth
Mr. Richard Clarke and Sam, Brother Heighes, and his two sons Sam and Bill,
Mr. and Mrs. White, and Mr. and Mrs. Pounsett dined, supped etc. there. We had a most elegant dinner, a whole Salmon, 3 boiled chicken and a Ham, a Neck of Mutton boiled with Capers, a green Goose rested and Peas, with Plumb Puddings and a Gooseberry Tart.

## Sept. 9
We had for dinner some common Fish, a Leg of Mutton rosted and a baked Pudding the first Course, and a rost Duck, a Meat Pye, Eggs and Tarts the second. For supper we had a brace of Partridges rosted, some cold Tongue, Potatoes in Shells and Tarts. I returned to Weston about past ten o'clock. To Servants at Ringland — 2. — gave o. 2. o. Mr. Custance also gave me to carry Home a brace of Partridges.

## Octob. 17
We had for dinner, the first Course, some Fish, Pike, a fine large piece of boiled Beef, Peas Soup, stewed Mutton, Goose Giblets, stewed etc. Second Course, a brace of Partridges, a Turkey rested, baked Pudding, Lobster, scolloped Oysters, and Tartlets. The desert black and white Grapes, Walnuts and small Nutts, Almonds and Raisins, Damson Cheese and Golden Pippms. Madeira, Lisbon, and Port Wines to drink.

# THE 1 SYSTEM

## Why are these diary excerpts relevant to a discussion about "The 1 System?"

Although Rev. Woodford probably understood at some level his penchant for gluttony wasn't healthy, he didn't have the nutritional knowledge or medical resources available to contemporary eaters. In short, WE KNOW BETTER.

We understand that excess weight is unhealthy. Readers of this book know far more than Rev. Woodford about cardiac problems and diabetes. We're all reasonably educated about good and bad fats, can generally recognize foods with high calorie content, have a fair understanding that complex carbohydrates are better than refined carbohydrates, and know far more than Rev. Woodford when it comes to lean meats, good oils, saturated fats, and consuming too much sugar.

We do know better. Some might say we don't have any valid excuses for not taking better care of ourselves.

In short, readers with gluttonous tendencies need to accept that gluttony is a problem. Once they've accepted and admitted that to themselves, "The 1 System" may offer help in overcoming those tendencies.

## ADD CANCER TO THE RISKS

> "Cardiac problems and diabetes are mentioned above. Those are real problems. So, too, is cancer. The multiple cancer risks associated with excess weight include breast, ovarian, prostate, and colon cancers; to name just a few."
>
> ~Harry L. Greene II MD

*"The 1 System" is all about developing common sense eating and motion habits.*

*The data are clear and undeniable.*

Moving your bones
will result in a healthier you.

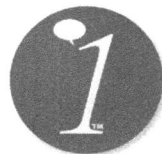

# IMPORTANT!
# CONSULT YOUR DOCTOR

## *1*

**Critical Rule**

*We cannot say this enough...*

It is important for you to consult a physician prior to embarking on any change in your dietary habits or exercise regimens; including "The 1 System."

We want all our readers to be as healthy as possible. Consulting with medical professionals cannot be overemphasized.

*Avoid the Scale!*

*The scale is not your friend.*

Keep your distance and only visit
that mass measuring device
1 Time a Month.

**A PERSONAL DRIFT WARNING**

"Modern cars now have an alarm to notify you when you are drifting out of your lane.

"A once a month weigh in can serve as a similar drift warning for you."

~Harry L. Greene II MD

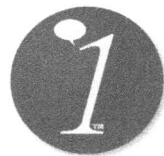

# WEIGHING YOURSELF

# 1
**Time Each Month**
**MAXIMUM**

Face it. Your weight gain occurred over a very long period of time. Yes, you can generally lose weight faster than you gained those unsightly pounds; regardless, it'll take a lot longer than you'd like. Get your arms around that and you'll have a greater chance of success.

Weight loss and gain are generally measured. We at "The 1 System" encourage you to avoid continually measuring your weight over short periods of time.

**Why?**
Weigh every day or two, and it can become depressing. Short term changes to your weight could be affected by the percentage of water in your body and the contents of your gastrointestinal tract, and not necessarily a reflection of the current state of fat cells in your body.

Weighing yourself once a week might show progress, but it can seed doubt and breed discouragement. Your weight was gained

## *Intended for Reader Use*

very slowly and moving to "The 1 System" may help you lose weight faster than you gained it, but losing weight is seldom on the same timetable as our hopes and expectations. Weighing once a month is sensible.

**AVOID OBSESSING**

"Don't be obsessive about weighing yourself. This is a life change."

~Harry L. Greene II MD

### 1st of the Month

We suggest you use the same date each month for weighing yourself. We like the number 1, as should you. You are Number 1 in our book about 1. We believe weighing yourself should occur 1 day a month, on day 1 of the month.

*It's all about*
## *"The Power of 1"*

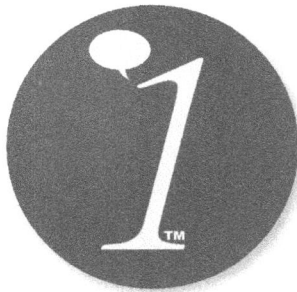

## Believing

*Desire, faith, or evidence?*

**A WEAK BELIEF**

> *"An empty approach, belief, and desire. As in,*
> *'I'm on a diet!'"*
> ~Harry L. Greene II MD

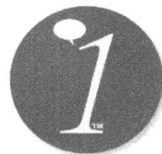

# BELIEF SYSTEMS

# 1

### Temporary Diet & My Weight Will Stabilize

Hoping a single temporary diet will stabilize your weight is just silly. It has no basis in fact and evidence. It's too weak to be considered a belief based on faith. It's more likely an empty desire.

**Most people believe a "Diet" is... TEMPORARY**
Unfortunately, the common contemporary use of the word "DIET" refers to a temporary modification of food and drink intake. More people would benefit if they seriously considered the long-term definition. "The 1 System's" goal is to assist you in focusing on long-term lifestyle habits and encourage avoidance of unhealthy short-term efforts to lose weight.

Studies indicate transient dieting usually results in weight gain, due to a decline of the body's metabolic rate; requiring less food to maintain stable body weight. That is precisely why most diets fail, and a return to normal eating habits will result in further weight gain.

Believe the facts.  Embrace the evidence.
**DIETS DON'T WORK!**

*Finally!*

*A Systematic Approach
That Really Works!*

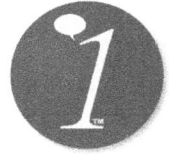

# THE 1 SYSTEM?

# 1

## Effective System To Address Eating Habits

This book is designed as an introduction to "The 1 System." In this book, we provide you with tools and information to assist you in modifying your lifestyle.

While we encourage readers to self-identify bad eating habits and find ways to overcome those bad habits, we also know the tactics, tips, tools, and tricks we developed can provide a logical, helpful foundation for anyone seeking lifestyle habit modification.

The following pages contain tactics, tips, tools, and tricks designed to assist you in modifying habits. Remember though, we are all different, and there's no single method available that will address everyone's needs. These approaches will need to be tailored to each person's individual needs. They are intended as guides only.

*Best wishes for success!*

# *Just Say*

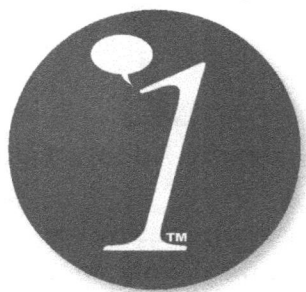

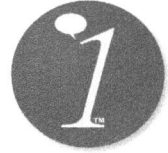

# PORTION CONTROL

# 1

### Reasonably Sized Portion, Per Item, Per Meal

Modern humans in first world countries gorge themselves regularly by heaping huge portions on their huge plates. If you consistently take reasonable portions and consume them slowly, you will, over time, become accustomed to smaller portions. In time, smaller portions should become habitual and satisfactory.

### KEY POINT:

*Make it a habit of serving yourself reasonably sized portions.*

### DARK HABITS

> "When to eat is also important. The same quantity of food, if eaten after dark, is more likely to be added as weight!"
>
> ~Harry L. Greene II MD

*Supersize Your Dinnerware?*

# *NOT!*

*Intended for Reader Use*

_____

_____

_____

_____

_____

_____

_____

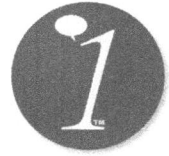

# PLATES, CUPS, GLASSES, & BOWLS

## 1
### Smaller Set of Dishware Items

**Plates**

It all starts with a single plate. People generally consume most of their food from a plate. Within mere minutes, we transfer the contents of the plate to our mouths. Moreover, we often refill that plate with additional and generally unnecessary food.

We believe it is both wise and critical to use smaller dish and utensil sizes; closer to those generally used in the 1960s and earlier. The plates you use should be no more than 6" to 8" in overall diameter; not the behemoth-sized plates used today.

Societal weight gain has grown steadily and parallel with the evolution of increasing plate sizes.

**Coffee Cups**

Many coffee cups are larger than a full cup. We recommend you use only cups that will hold a single measured cup of fluid.

# STEVEN FOWLER

*Intended for Reader Use*

**Drinking Glasses**
Do you really need 12 and 16 fluid ounce glasses in your kitchen? In most cases, if someone fills a glass with a beverage, they're usually going to fill it to the top. Why drink 16 ounces of milk when you would have been satisfied with 8 ounces. Ditch the larger vessels and downsize your drinking glasses to 8 fluid ounces (1 cup) maximum.

If you insist on keeping and using 12 and 16 ounce glasses, consider using them only for water and unsweetened tea.

**Bowls**
As with plates, bowls have also expanded over time. We suggest you fill your cereal bowl with water, then pour it into a measuring cup. Many bowls sold today will easily hold a full pint of water (2 cups). We suggest you use a bowl no larger than a ½ pint (1 cup).

### DEVELOP THIS HABIT

"Try having a cup of soup, rather than a bowl. You'll hardly notice the difference."

~Harry L. Greene II MD

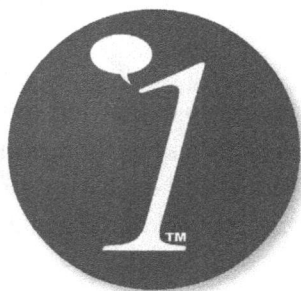

STEVEN FOWLER

*The Power of 1!*

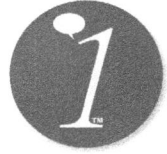

# IT'S ALL ABOUT THE 1'S

## 1
### Can Be Your Best Friend

This is the part of the book where we launch into "The 1's."

1's are guidelines that can help usher you down a path toward better living. It's all about taking control of your life, modifying your habits, and remaining conscious of what you do with your body.

### Day at a Time
New habits take time to develop

Remember, life is lived 1 day at a time. Expecting long-lived habits to change in a few days, weeks, or months is unrealistic and downright silly.

*Intended for Reader Use*

_____

_____

_____

_____

_____

_____

_____

_____

_____

_____

_____

_____

_____

_____

_____

_____

_____

_____

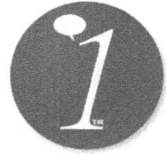

# SHARE YOUR ONES

## 1
### Thing About Sharing

As 1's are shared, others will benefit. You might share a single 1 and benefit dozens, hundreds, or more.
*You never know. You may unknowingly help save a life.*

On the other hand, you might be the beneficiary of someone sharing a single "1" that will propel you to success as you follow "The 1 System."

Have you discovered a 1 in your life that you'd like to share? *Great!* Use the form at:

www.The1System.com

That simple form is designed to share your 1's with others. This author and the publisher will consolidate the best 1's received and include them in the second book of this series. We hope to publish that book in late 2019.

**Effective Submission Might Save A Life!**

# STEVEN FOWLER

*Intended for Reader Use*

_____

_____

_____

_____

_____

_____

_____

_____

_____

_____

_____

_____

_____

_____

_____

_____

_____

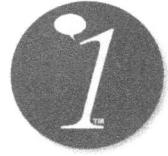

# GENERAL ONES

### Simple Approach to Dieting
Just Count to 1

This is wonderfully easy. You don't count calories or need to count points. You don't have to open a box that came in the mail and heat it up. None of those things. All you have to do is remember a number: 1

### Pound at a Time
Don't get in a hurry!

Goals are important, but setting high expectations for quick achievement with difficult goals is dangerous. If you decided to walk from Los Angeles to New York, you wouldn't expect to accomplish the feat in a week or two. Just so, be realistic about your weight.

Getting to New York from the west coast is accomplished 1 step at a time. No more. Likewise, losing twenty or thirty pounds is accomplished 1 pound at a time.

# STEVEN FOWLER

## *Intended for Reader Use*

_____

_____

_____

_____

_____

_____

_____

_____

_____

_____

_____

_____

_____

_____

_____

_____

Approach goal setting in this manner. What does it matter if you only lose 3 pounds in a month? At that rate, in a year, you will lose nearly 40 pounds.

After all, if you need to lose 40 pounds, I would bet it took most of you many years to accumulate that weight. You didn't gain it overnight, so don't expect to lose it overnight.

"Gee, I only lost 2 pounds all week! I give up!"

*Do you talk like that? Do you say such things?*

Let's do some math. 2 pounds times 52 weeks in a year equals - WOW! 104 Pounds!

Look at the big picture, your long-range goals, and for goodness sake, stay off the scale!

Worry about your consumption and activities. The weight will take care of itself. Too many people spend too much time worrying about today's pound. Focus on food intake, not your weight.

**Serving**
Easy to remember

The practice of returning for second and third servings is commonplace and detrimental. Don't refill your plate. A single serving is normally sufficient for your nutritional needs, if your diet is well balanced and supplemented with a good multivitamin.

1's are easy to remember. *1 Serving – Period!*

This isn't The 2 System, The 3 System, or The 4 System.

# STEVEN FOWLER

*Intended for Reader Use*

### ① Small Meal 4 Times Each Day
Start Early and Eat Often

Regular eating habits are essential to good health and weight management. We suggest you eat four small meals each day. Many people skip breakfast as part of their daily eating habits. Others insist breakfast is important.

There's one school of thought that consuming food early in the day kicks your metabolic rate upward and, in layman's terms, gets your calorie-burning fires going. Some of that thinking is based on a study reported to have been funded by a cereal company.

Another unproven theory is that failing to eat breakfast slows your metabolism and encourages your body to gain weight; not to mention the adverse effects that failing to eat might have on your blood sugar levels.

We believe eating reasonably in the morning is good for most people, when food choices are carefully considered. We don't believe it is prudent to begin the day with sugary fattening foods like most cold cereals, granola (take a look at the ingredients), sweetened yogurt, sweet pastries, donuts, most breakfast bars, orange juice (eat an orange instead), and other desserts for breakfast.

Yes, I said desserts. Simply put, many breakfast choices, based on the ingredients, are best described as desserts.

The same can be said for many commercially available coffee drinks prepared by your favorite barista. Syrup and chocolate laden coffee beverages, covered with whipped cream are little more than caffeinated milk shakes.

---

## "DON'T EAT AFTER SUPPER!"
~Harry L. Greene II MD

---

*Intended for Reader Use*

# THE 1 SYSTEM

**Reasonably Sized Portion**
Per Item. Per Meal.

Modern Americans gorge themselves regularly by heaping huge portions on their plates. If you consistently take reasonable portions and consume them slowly, you will, over time, become accustomed to smaller portions. In time, smaller portions should become habitual and satisfying.

**Fist-Sized Portion**

A rule of thumb approach to portion size offered by more than a few nutritionists is to limit any given portion to the size of your own fist. We don't believe this will, necessarily, work for all people. However, if you're currently eating portions larger than your fist, this would be a good option to embrace on your way to a healthier you. If, over time, you find a fist-sized portion is a larger size than you need, then make the adjustments necessary to meet your needs.

**Small Food-Grade Scale**

Some may find value by using a small food-grade scale as they work to make adjustments to their own needs under "The 1 System."

If you're so inclined, use a scale to weigh what you're eating and keep a record of food items consumed and the weight involved. Over time you can determine if you need to adjust the quantities involved to meet your goals.

# STEVEN FOWLER

*Intended for Reader Use*

---

**Glass of Water**
15 Minutes Before Each Meal

This doesn't mean you need to stretch your stomach with 16 ounces of water. Four to six ounces will serve you well.

Some might ask if water is all that important. Here's a chemistry joke that very well answers that question:

## If H₂O is water, what is H₂O₄?

Drinking, bathing, sailing, dieting, and more...

**Glass of Water**
15 Minutes After Each Meal

**Percent Milk will Reduce Caloric Intake**

**Food and Exercise Journal**

Studies demonstrate weight loss and weight management is more successful for those who record their eating and exercise activities.

If you choose to record in a journal, we at "The 1 System" suggest you consider adding a number to what you eat. Use a "1" if what you ate was within your plan for using "The 1 System." If you went beyond your planned "1" you can determine if what you consumed was twice, three times, or more than you should have eaten under your plan.

# STEVEN FOWLER

*Intended for Reader Use*

_____

_____

_____

_____

_____

_____

_____

_____

_____

_____

_____

_____

_____

_____

When looking back at your journal, if you see mostly "1's" give yourself a pat on the back. You're probably well on your way to success with "The 1 System." If you see "2's" "3's" and "4's" you should do some real soul searching. Redouble your efforts to set new, reasonable, achievable goals.

## ① Glass of Wine

If you drink wine, we recommend you consume red wine. Use a reasonably sized glass. Studies indicate the benefits associated with a single glass of red wine outweigh the benefits of white wine.

Most people are aware of the studies suggesting a glass of red wine each day is heart healthy. However, some people take it to heart in unhealthy ways and consume too many glasses. Stop at 1 glass.

## ① Alcoholic Beverage Per Day MAXIMUM

If you drink alcoholic beverages other than wine or beer, we recommend you avoid sweetened mixes.

# STEVEN FOWLER

## *Intended for Reader Use*

# **1** Calorie Soda

We suggest you limit the intake of diet sodas to 1 per day. There are several reasons for this approach.

First, artificial sweeteners really aren't good for humans. For most, limiting intake of these sweeteners to a single soda each day shouldn't be a problem.

Second, ingesting artificial sweeteners seems to play a role in limiting the ability to lose weight in a number of popular contemporary diets.

Third, artificial sweeteners remind your body that sweet exists. Reducing your intake of artificial and natural sweeteners reduces your craving for sweets.

Have you ever wondered if the human stomach is designed to accommodate those gigantic 32 ounce sodas you often see people carrying?

Have you noticed there's a common body type associated with those you see carrying large soft drink and sweet coffee drink containers? Very often, the larger the container, the larger the person. Many of those people are seldom seen without a beverage in their hands.

We believe anyone who must carry a drink in hand at all times would be wise to choose WATER.

Plain old water. Non-flavored, non-sweetened, $H_2O$.

# STEVEN FOWLER

## *Intended for Reader Use*

_____

_____

_____

_____

_____

_____

_____

_____

_____

_____

_____

_____

_____

_____

_____

## **1** Regular Soda Per Week
This should be considered a Treat Item.

If you feel you must consume sugary beverages, we heartily suggest you limit the intake of sugared sodas to: 1 per week – MAXIMUM!

*Better yet, 1 per month.*
We recognize the treat value in sodas. Therefore we suggest you tightly restrict the consumption of sodas. There are several reasons for this approach.

First, refined sugar (regardless of the name, e.g., fructose) really isn't good for you.

Second, reducing your intake of natural sweeteners reduces your craving for sweets.

Third, sweets retard your ability to lose weight.

While we suggest you stop drinking sodas entirely, we recognize this might hinder your ability to maintain your involvement with "The 1 System."

### A TASTY ALTERNATIVE

"Try using a lemon flavored non-sugared soda."
~Harry L. Greene II MD

# STEVEN FOWLER

*Intended for Reader Use*

_____

_____

_____

_____

_____

_____

_____

_____

_____

_____

_____

_____

_____

_____

_____

_____

If you choose this Treat Item, make certain you only purchase and keep 1 treat beverage in your home per week or month. If you only have 1 in stock, it will continually remind you that, once it is gone, there isn't a second beverage available. That may assist you to hold off drinking it until you find a special occasion that will justify using the final soda in the house.

Over time, it's likely you'll find your interest in that sweet drink is waning.

### 1 Cup of Black Coffee Per Day

Black. Avoid creams and sugars. If you already use one or both, those need to become a much smaller part of your life.

1 cup is all about reducing your consumption across the board.

### 1 Fewer, 1 Less, 1 Smaller
Use your imagination

You're familiar with the 1 slice fewer method I employed to downsize my pizza consumption. An approach of that type can be used by followers of "The 1 System" in many ways.

For example, followers who enjoy a large barista-prepared sweetened, and/or fat-filled, coffee concoction each morning and afternoon can modify that habit in many positive ways. If a follower pledges to begin drinking the same beverage, but drops from the extra-large version to

*Intended for Reader Use*

the large version for an entire week, they'll not only reduce fat, calorie, and sugar intake, they'll save money in the process.

After a week they might decide to drop from large to the medium size, and so forth. Then adjust further by dedicating that afternoon trip to the coffee bar for a black coffee or sugar-free beverage (e.g., tea). After making that helpful adjustment, and allowing a short reasonable period of time to pass, further adjust further by modifying that morning cream-filled syrupy whipped cream-laden drink, to something more healthy.

Perhaps they can go a week without the whipped cream. After another week that person might decide it is time to forgo the syrup. Coffee and cream only. In another week the cream might be removed as well.

This author believes in a "boiling the frog" approach to lifestyle modification. Slowly change, like slowing raising the temperature in a frog-filled pot of water, and you will scarcely notice or miss what has been left behind.

Ease into a system of your own design, using "The Power of 1." There's nothing like that most excellent feeling enjoyed by successful followers when they see a photo someone took from behind, and realize some of their own behind has been left behind.

## NEEDS BASED MULTIVITAMINS

"Vitamins are often formulated based on needs across the age spectrum (e.g., Centrum Silver Adult 50+)."
~Harry L. Greene II MD

# STEVEN FOWLER

*Intended for Reader Use*

_____

_____

_____

_____

_____

_____

_____

_____

_____

_____

_____

_____

_____

_____

_____

# The 1 System

## 1 Daily Multivitamin

Most adults will benefit from taking a daily multivitamin. We urge you to consult with your family physician abouttaking a supplemental multivitamin as part of your daily approach to "The 1 System."

## 1 Potato Dish Per Week
This should be considered a Treat Item.

Garlic Mashed Potatoes, French Fries, Au Gratin Potatoes, Baked Potato, etc... The list goes on.

Pick a day, keep the quantity down, chew slowly, chew completely, and savor every bite. Avoid adding quantities of butter, ketchup, cheeses, sour cream, and other fat laden and sugary condiments to your potato. If it doesn't taste good to you all by itself, consider whether you really want and need a potato dish.

## 1 Deep Fried Serving Per Week
(e.g., French fries, fish, fried chicken, etc...)

If you're keeping your potato intake to 1 per week, this deep fried option will qualify as meeting your quota for BOTH your potato AND fried food serving.

# STEVEN FOWLER

*Intended for Reader Use*

### ① Weekly Scoop of Ice Cream
*No Sugar Added is Best*

Ice cream is filled with fat, sugars, and other items that make it taste great, but also add girth to your body and plaque in your arteries. For many, ice cream is a wonderful addition to their dietary intake. A treat, if you will.

We recognize the importance of the enjoyment gained by enjoying dessert items like ice cream and suggest you keep the intake of this treat to a minimum. While we don't believe you should necessarily deny yourself the pleasure of this wonderful concoction, we recommend you approach eating ice cream in moderation. Consume ice cream no more than once a week and limit your intake to a single reasonably sized scoop. 1 time a month would be even better. In some cases, gelato might be a better alternative to ice cream.

**PUT IT DOWN**

> "Force yourself to taste the food by putting the fork down after each bite."
>
> ~Harry L. Greene II MD

# STEVEN FOWLER

*Intended for Reader Use*

**Habit You Should Develop**
It's all about the digestive process.

**Chew Until Liquefied**

I'll watch others chew with amazement. Some people will take a bite of something and chew it two or three times before swallowing. *Masticating is important!* Masticating?

Yes, masticating means chewing. We have teeth designed for biting, tearing, chewing, and grinding. The digestive process actively begins when we bite into our food. The salivary glands go to work as we chew and begin breaking down the food in our mouths. A good rule of thumb to assist in the process is to chew until every bite is liquefied before swallowing.

Yesterday I was sitting at a long stoplight. A pickup truck pulled alongside me. I watched in disbelief as a young man consumed a huge (high and wide), 2 or 3 patty, loaded cheeseburger in 3 bites.

He chewed the first massive bite in exactly 3 chews. Bites 2 and 3 required 5 chews each. 13 chews total for that giant burger!

*NOT GOOD!*

*Bite at a Time*
*Savor every single bite you take.*

Have you ever caught yourself eating without thinking; without enjoying the tastes filling your mouth? Why shovel calories down your throat without thought or satisfaction if you're trying to manage your weight?

# STEVEN FOWLER

## *Intended for Reader Use*

_____

_____

_____

_____

_____

_____

_____

_____

_____

_____

_____

_____

_____

_____

_____

**1 Liquid Meal Each Day**
During the first month.

We believe it is important to start "The 1 System" by reducing your cravings and addressing your stomach's desire to fill and stretch. Try to make 1 of your meals, for the first month, a liquid-based meal. Soup is a good choice. No, you don't have to have bread, butter, tortillas, crackers or other "outside the bowl" items with your soup. Soup only. 1 cup.

The preferred meal for this approach is dinner. Yes, you may find yourself a little less satisfied for a few days, but this is an important first step if you'd like to jump start your efforts to modify your habits.

If your soup is purchased from a store, make certain it is low sodium and low fat. Purchase soups that are made using a water foundation, as opposed to a milk, cream, or similar.

If possible, it is always better to make your own soup. There are many good, tasty, satisfying, and healthy soup recipes available online.

**1 Low Carb (Lite) Alcoholic Beer Per Day**

Are you someone who enjoys a cold beer, or two, or three, or more? If so, consuming a single low carbohydrate bottle of suds will give you the tasty pleasure you enjoy, without suffering the various problems associated with drinking

# STEVEN FOWLER

*Intended for Reader Use*

_____

_____

_____

_____

_____

_____

_____

_____

_____

_____

_____

_____

_____

_____

_____

_____

_____

multiple beers each day.

Do you drink every day? Take it to the next level, and skip 1 day after drinking 1 beer. Then repeat the pattern. After a while you might consider graduating to 1 beer a week; while savoring every swallow.

Of course, graduate level beer drinking might mean 1 beer a month. *There's power in the Power of 1!*

## ① Candy

I love chocolate covered peanuts. When my wife and I were younger, we'd go to the movies with our friends Mark and Pam. Tracey and I would consume a giant bag of those wonderful treats (provided by Pam). We still enjoy them once or twice a week, but not the whole bag. We'll each eat a single candy and savor every second of it. At that point we're satisfied. We don't deny ourselves, nor do we pig out on the tasty treats.

## ① Support Person Is Helpful

Most people benefit from the encouragement of others. Moreover, those who've traveled an identical path at some time in the past, or are willing to travel that path with you now, are more likely to help you in your quest. Find at least 1 support person to assist and encourage you with Steven Fowler's "The 1 System."

# STEVEN FOWLER

*Intended for Reader Use*

_____

_____

_____

_____

_____

_____

_____

_____

_____

_____

_____

_____

_____

_____

_____

_____

There's no question. Having a support person will help you achieve success in the habit modification arena. If you offer that person a measure of trust, transparency, and accountability - the chances of achieving your goals will increase exponentially.

**① Meal Should Take No Less Than 15 Minutes to Eat**
The slower you go, the faster you'll feel full.

Want to see something eye opening and helpful in your quest to gain control of your weight? Have your support person secretly videotape you at home and in restaurants. Most of us don't realize just how awful we look as we pack food into the upper end of our digestive tract. *Yuck!*

Consider this. It's not just you. Next time you're in a restaurant pay attention (without staring) to just how long it takes for people to clean their plates. It's absolutely amazing how quickly food can disappear. Some can make their food vanish without even chewing.

### FORK DOWN AND DRINK

"As mentioned previously, put the fork down between bites. Take a drink of water too."

~Harry L. Greene II MD

# STEVEN FOWLER

*Intended for Reader Use*

### ① Item From Each Food Group Each Day

Try to eat at least 1 item from each food group during at least 1 of your daily meals. Remember to keep your portions small.

### ① Day at a Time

Remember, life is lived 1 day at a time. New habits take more than 1 day to develop. Learn and practice patience.

### ① Slice of Pizza
*Don't forget, 1 slice at a time led
to the discovery of "The Power of 1."*

Shortly after I began to develop "The 1 System," I realized my bad eating habits weren't restricted to pizza. I love corn tortillas, covered with cheese, melted in a microwave oven, and finished off with habanero pepper sauce.

Using one of our ginormous dinner plates, I'd place 4 corn tortillas around the plate (nearly covering the entire surface), then pile shredded cheese across the tortillas. Once melted and spiced up with hot sauce, I'd gobble them down, THEN repeat the entire process one or more times.

I tried going cold turkey and dropping down to a single tortilla, but found I wasn't satisfied. Then I decided to do the same thing I did with pizza. Over the next few weeks, I

*Intended for Reader Use*

began using 1 less tortilla each time I prepared that "snack," until I was down to cooking and eating 1 cheese-covered tortilla at a time. That's all I eat now. Just 1.

Smokers know some people can stop smoking cold turkey and others find they need to slowly decrease the number of cigarettes smoked over a  period of time.

Find what works for you, then fold it into your plan to achieve your goals. You may find slowly decreasing everything is best for you. On the other hand, some find find it easier to jump headlong into going cold turkey. Even others may find additional tweaks to get them there, using a combination of approaches. The good doctor offers one such approach, by going smaller as part of the equation:

## THE INCREDIBLE SHRINKING TORTILLA

> "Go from a 12" tortilla, to a 6" or 8" tortilla."
> ~Harry L. Greene II MD

Likewise, some of you will need to slowly decrease consumption, while others can successfully drop to their established goal right away.

# STEVEN FOWLER

*Intended for Reader Use*

_____

_____

_____

_____

_____

_____

_____

_____

_____

_____

_____

_____

_____

_____

_____

_____

**1 Glass of Almond Milk**
Less calories than dairy.

Cow's milk weighs in at 150 calories per 8 ounces.

Same Quantity: Unsweetened Almond Milk = 40 calories.

**1 Bite of Dessert**
*Since when did dessert become a meal?*

Savor, relish, and enjoy. A single bite tastes the same as eating ten or more bites, right? It's about the taste, not the nourishment or quantity. Therefore, take 1 bite and enjoy it like it's twenty. *Ah… The Power of 1!*

**1 Calorie Gum**

**1 Calorie Salad Dressing**

**1 Mile Covered Each Day**

Walk, bike, or run, it doesn't matter. Just move your body, your bones. If you can go farther, do so.

*Intended for Reader Use*

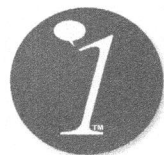

# EATING OUT

## Restaurant Meal Per Week

Restaurants are notorious for serving high calorie meals. Many of these meals are prepared with too much salt, sugar, and fat. Americans eat many more meals at restaurants than we did only a generation or two ago. In that time, our average body weight has increased.

Many restaurants want you to feel like you received your money's worth, so they load you up with huge portions of high fat, high calorie, and high sodium foods. Such meals leave you less than satisfied, bloated, and they super size your waistline.

## Meal for Two People
*Ask for an additional plate**

This can be a Win-Win for two people. Split your meal, while saving money and calories.

Eating alone? Splitting isn't an option? No worries. Ask the server to bring you a doggie bag when the food is delivered. Split your meal when it arrives and save the other half for later.

# STEVEN FOWLER

*Intended for Reader Use*

_____

_____

_____

_____

_____

_____

_____

_____

_____

_____

_____

_____

_____

_____

_____

*Note: Some restaurants will upcharge the meal if you ask for an additional plate. The good doctor offers an excellent solution for this situation. Moreover, even if the restaurant doesn't levy an upcharge for an additional plate, Dr. Greene's solution will work equally well.*

## WHAT'S MINE IS YOURS

"1 person can order the main course, and the other can order a salad. Then both plates can be split and shared between the two persons."

~Harry L. Greene II MD

### Fast Food Visit Per Week

Many readers would be surprised to know how many people eat at fast food establishments multiple times each week. Fast food restaurants are famous for serving up loads of high calorie, high sodium, fatty meals. While some of my readers have little interest in fast food fare, many do.

### Item Per Order at the Restaurant
No Appetizer. Dessert.

Plan your restaurant ordering carefully. Avoid costly appetizers and desserts (save $$$ & calories). Find the

*Intended for Reader Use*

items on the menu you enjoy eating. Then look at which one best suits your desire to improve your eating habits. Choose that item.

Denying oneself will often lead to failure in reader efforts to modify your dietary habits. Order what you want, within reason. Whatever you do, don't order out of habit; until and unless you've developed GOOD eating habits. Order out of conviction and enjoyment.

*Don't order out of habit.*
*Do save your hard earned money, so don't order appetizers.*
*Do save your waistline, so don't order desserts.*

**1 Page, 1 Bite**
Read 1 page, take 1 bite.

Do you read when you eat? If so, be careful. Don't forget to savor your meal. While doing so, try this. Eat 1 bite, savor every chew, swallow, sip some water, read a page, then (and only then) enjoy another bite.

*Intended for Reader Use*

_____

_____

_____

_____

_____

_____

_____

_____

_____

_____

_____

_____

_____

_____

_____

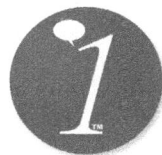

# CHALLENGE ITEMS

### Action Item for You to Adopt
*Stop the silliness.*

We all see people blocking parking lot aisles, trying to gain access to a parking space near the front door; when a perfectly good space is located 15 or 20 feet farther away.

I recently watched a lady I know go around, and around, and around a parking lot trying to get a spot closer to the door. She eventually acquired a spot about a 100' closer by driving in circles.

Later, when she exited the store, I approached her and had a nice visit. At one point I looked down and noticed an exercise tracker on her wrist. I asked if she calculated how far she walked inside the store. She said she did and proudly told me ¼ mile and the number of steps she took.

Why does someone drive in circles to save a 100' feet on a beautiful day, then go inside and walk many times that distance? *Do they realize others are watching them in disbelief and amusement?*

We suggest followers of "The 1 System" become selfish when it comes to parking lots. Think of yourself first. Park as far away as possible to increase your opportunities to move your body just a little more. Be selfish and let chubby people park near the door.

## *Intended for Reader Use*

_____

_____

_____

_____

_____

_____

_____

_____

_____

_____

_____

_____

_____

_____

_____

_____

THE 1 SYSTEM

### ① Recommendation for Costco Shoppers

Next time you visit Costco, park as far from the main entrance as possible. Enter the store and make 1 pass only at the snack tables. Consider skipping the sweet samples and processed food samples. *Enjoy!* Then shop.

By then you might be less hungry, and some of those unnecessary impulse purchases may fail to materialize.

### ① Flight = 1 Snack

On a flight? Flight attendants will often toss you two or more bags of peanuts or other snacks. If you really want the snack, fine (at least the portions are small). Just eat 1 and give away the second.

Alternatively, you can save the second for later or leave it with your trash. Regardless, don't eat the second snack on the same flight as the first.

This author occasionally relies on a single tablespoon of light yogurt to accomplish what the good doctor suggests below.

### ADDRESSING HUNGER

"Snack on something like Yoplait Light (very small servings), between meals when hungry!"
~Harry L. Greene II MD

# STEVEN FOWLER

*Intended for Reader Use*

_____

_____

_____

_____

_____

_____

_____

_____

_____

_____

_____

_____

_____

_____

_____

_____

_____

## ①  Meal Daily with Chopsticks

Eating meals with chopsticks will generally result in longer eating times and feeling a sensation of fullness before you've eaten too much.

## ①  Must Not Get Too Hungry
Gorging isn't good!

Try to avoid going too long between meals. It may result in you getting too hungry and losing sight of "The 1 System" on that occasion. I should know. I'm very familiar with this problem. If I become too hungry I catch myself pigging out. This is a problem I continually work to overcome. The best medicine I've found is to avoid getting too famished.

## ①  Circular Pattern at the Grocery Store

Eat healthier, consume less fat, sodium, and sugar by avoiding grocery store aisles. Sweets, refined carbs, and heavily processed foods dominate interior aisles.

Try doing the majority, if not all, of your grocery shopping by remaining out the outer perimeter of the store. Fresh vegetables, the deli, the meat counter, dairy, and brown breads inhabit the periphery of most grocery stores.

# STEVEN FOWLER

*Intended for Reader Use*

---

---

---

---

---

---

---

---

---

---

---

---

---

---

---

### ① Tactic, Tip, Tool, or Trick a Day

Write, review, iterate, review, succeed and celebrate.

Spend time daily trying to adapt "The 1 System" into your life, and record what you've come up with to improve your chances to enjoy success with "The 1 System." By extension, we believe if you do well in this area, your goals will be more achievable.

Use the lined real estate provided in the pages of this book, and benefit from your handiwork.

# STEVEN FOWLER

*Intended for Reader Use*

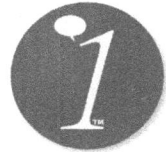

# EXPECTATIONS

### Very Important Rule
*Keep your expectations reasonable.*

If you raise your expectations, requirements, and goals too high, you are doomed to fail. Your eating and exercise habits were developed over many years and attempting to modify them over an unrealistically brief period will breed certain failure for most people.

### A HEALTHY PERSPECTIVE

"Remember, a slip is not a fall!"
~Harry L. Greene II MD

# STEVEN FOWLER

*Intended for Reader Use*

_____

_____

_____

_____

_____

_____

_____

_____

_____

_____

_____

_____

_____

_____

_____

_____

120

**Size at a Time**

### Ladies
Contentment should come with shrinking 1 dress size at a time. Set reasonable goals and adjust your 1's reasonably, if the next lower dress size remains elusive after a reasonable period of time.

### Men
Gentlemen, like the ladies, you need to keep your clothes size reduction goals modest and reasonable. Don't think you're going to drop from a 48" waist to a 36" waist overnight. Be happy with moving to another notch on your belt over a period of months; not days or weeks.

*Intended for Reader Use*

### It's Your Turn

*We've laid the foundation;*
*the rest is up to you.*

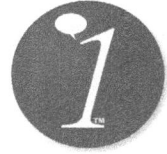

# THE CHALLENGE

# *1*

## More Thing

Now that you're in possession of "The 1 System's" introductory tactics, tips, tools, and tricks (4T's), we want to challenge you to succeed in achieving your goals.

Any modification of your habits is entirely up to you. We've provided you with some starting 4T's for your "Personal 1 System." Plant those seeds and develop more. Create "Seeds of 1" for further planting and development. Here's where you tailor "The 1 System" to your own needs.

For example, if you believe eating 1 Slice of Toast in the morning is too much for you, but you don't want to do without. *Great!* Modify your "Personal 1 System" from 1 Slice of Toast to ½ Slice of Toast.

Tailor "The 1 System" to your needs. Everyone is different. Some might find they've lost more weight than desired with the existing 1's. They might decide 1 potato a week isn't enough. In that case they might adjust and make it 1 potato dish twice a week.

# STEVEN FOWLER

*Intended for Reader Use*

Along the way, as you come up with 4T's of your own, we'd appreciate you sharing. If enough "1's" and other tips are offered by readers, the next book will contain the 1's deemed best for sharing with others. You will be credited in a manner similar to that shown below.

**Small Milkshake Once A Month**
A Treat Item.

1 small milkshake only as a Treat Item, 1 time a month.
Joan P.
Land 'O Lakes, WI

Submissions can sent to us via "The 1 System" website.

www.The1System.com

Thank you in advance for your submissions.

*NOTE: All submissions must be submitted without license, restrictions, or expectations of remuneration. All submissions will pass freely to Two Loons Press and shall not be encumbered in any manner whatsoever. Submissions may be used by Two Loons Press online, in printed form, downloaded into eBooks, or in other ways. Neither the author nor the publisher will be held responsible for payment of any kind relating to submissions.*

STEVEN FOWLER

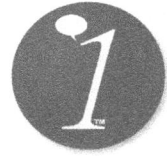

# ABOUT THE AUTHOR

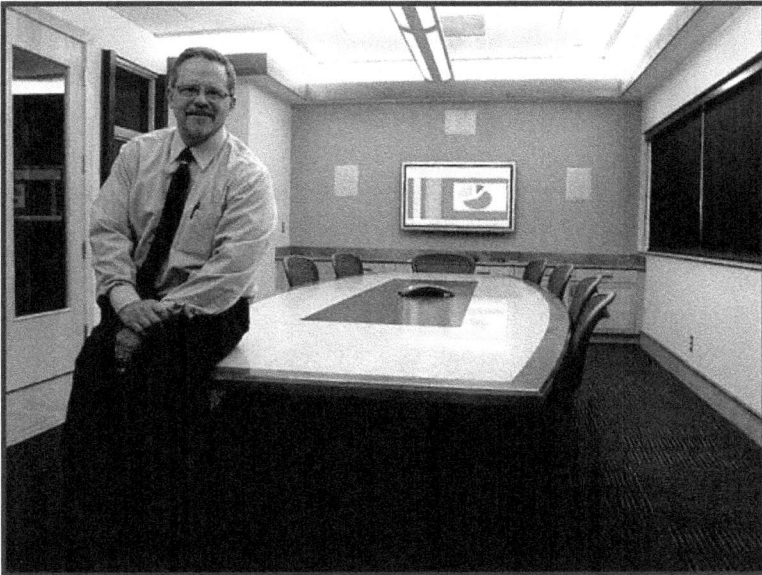

Steven Fowler, and his wife Tracey, reside in Oro Valley, Arizona.

Tracey works in education. Their daughter serves as a police dispatcher with a law enforcement agency, and their U.S. Marine son, a combat veteran, is in training to become a commercial airline pilot. Each are married to two wonderful people and, as of this writing, have blessed Steven and Tracey with 4 grandchildren.

Mr. Fowler is a semi-retired entrepreneur and corporate executive, who dedicates his free time to pursue his passion as a writer. He writes in pursuit of pleasure, charitable causes, and for various business purposes.

# WHEN?

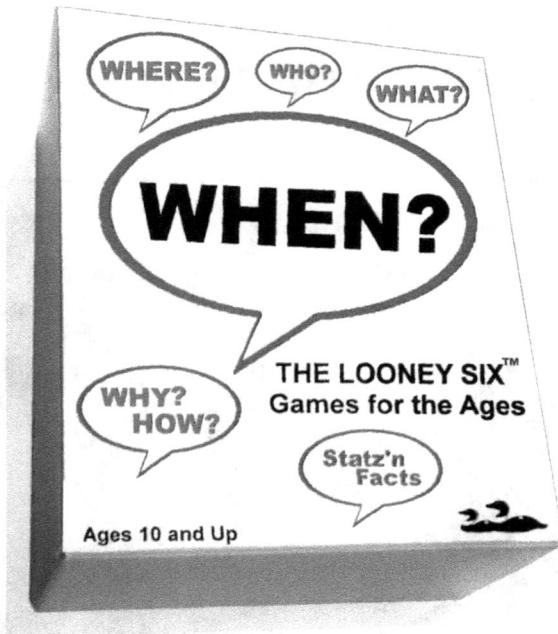

A history-inspired game for ages 10 and up.
2 or More Players
2 or More Teams

Don't like or know history?
Doesn't Matter

Guessing, Figuring, and Knowing
are all part of the game.

Scheduled for Release in the U.S. and Canada
FALL 2019

Steven Fowler is also the inventor of "The Looney Six™" Game Series.

"**WHEN?**, a game built upon culture, sports, entertainment, invention, political, and other history-inspired people, places, and events. **WHEN?** involves guessing, figuring, and recollection for ages 10 and up, involving 2 or more people or teams. Knowledge, logic, deductive reasoning, and some basic math can propel one team to victory, or not.

**WHEN?** is currently undergoing beta and market testing. It is scheduled for a Fall 2019 release by Two Loons Press. **WHEN?** is expected to be available online and in retail locations throughout the U.S. and Canada.

Other games in "The Looney Six™" Game Series are scheduled for release in the coming years.

## "The Looney Six™" Game Series will include the following games:

- **WHO?**
- **WHAT?**
- **WHERE?**
- **WHEN?**
- **WHY & HOW?**
- **Statz 'n Facts!**

This author and Two Loons Press wish you the very best on your journey with the "The 1 System."

*"The 1 System," a lifestyle diet centered around 1 (you)!*

# Have Fun
# with

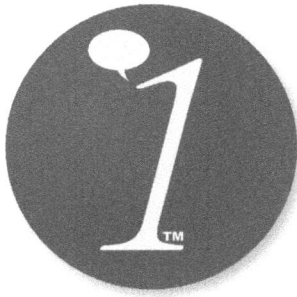

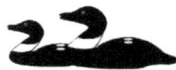

TWO LOONS PRESS

www.ingramcontent.com/pod-product-compliance
Lightning Source LLC
Chambersburg PA
CBHW050348280326
41933CB00010BA/1380